Sex Positions:

Top 10 Unusual Sex Positions +20 Ways To Find the G-Spot

Table of content

Introduction

I want to thank and congratulate you on downloading **"Sex: Top 10 Sex Positions for Astonishing Sex and Proven Methods to Find G-spot."** Within the pages of this book you will find proven steps and strategies on how you can keep the passion heated in the bedroom. You will be introduced to ten top sexual positions that are guaranteed to help you to accomplish results where you have your sexual partner begging for more as they twist and shout with pleasure.

Once you have read this book you will have mastered these top ten sexual positions in theory. The next step beyond that is to take these new learned positions and apply them to your repertoire and make your partner begging for you to sexually please them again and again using your new learned techniques that are going to add some spice and excitement to your love life!

Chapter 1 – Different Approaches to the Missionary Style

In this chapter we are taking a look at some different approaches to the missionary style that will help add some new spark to your lovemaking.

The Dirty Dangle

This is a different take on the missionary position that involves the woman lying on her back near the edge of the bed. You will enjoy this lovemaking session. As you are getting close to your climax, slowly inch toward the foot of the bed until the woman has her head over the edge of the bed and her arms are hanging over the edge of the bed. Her arms can touch the floor while her head hangs back. The man should continue thrusting until they reach orgasm. The rush about this position is the feeling the woman gets with the blood rushing to her head at the same time as she is climaxing. Sex experts label this sensation as "erotic inversion." The woman will have a different orgasmic experience because she has the feeling that she is upside down. This is not a position recommended for those that tend to suffer from light-headedness.

The Pillow Driver

This is another variation of the missionary position, the use of a pillow will be necessary. While the woman is lying on her back prop her butt up using a pillow or two. Her knees should be bent up while her legs are wide apart. Place her arms above her head or at the man's sides. The man then gets on top of the woman with his hands placed on either side of bed or floor at the woman's head. This will cause him to penetrate the vagina at a higher angle than usual. As the man is moving he must perform a push-like motion using his hands to control his weight and avoid pinning down his partner underneath him. He should use slow moving thrusts so that his female partner can feel his manhood. The pillows allow for deeper penetration which can help stimulate the clitoris more. The man can vary his movements to keep his female partner feeling different sensations. One motion to help induce orgasm is using the figure-eight. The man draws the figure-eight using hip movements. This movement will help to stimulate the vagina more and allows the pubic bone to stimulate the clitoris.

Before the man enters the woman with his penis he can lube up the woman using his tongue and giving her some oral sex. With her pelvis propped on on the pillows this will expose her clitoris even more, making it ready for some oral sex before penetration with the penis.

Clitty Cat

The Clitty Cat is one of the best sex positions that deviates a bit from the missionary style. The missionary style is one of the classic positions, but even this can become boring when done over and over again in the same way. If you have a routine like way of lovemaking it can lead to a boring sex life. This in turn can lead to having problems in the relationship. The Cat in the Clitty Cat stands for "Coital Alignment Technique." The renowned sex researcher Edward Eichel first introduced this position in 1988 after he discovered that just by making a simple adjustment to the missionary position would allow women to enjoy lovemaking even more. With the Cat position it allows for more clitoral contact. Many women who had had problems obtaining an orgasm found that when they tried the Clitty Cat technique they were able to reach orgasm. It was even stated in the Journal of Sex and Martial Therapy that women were 56% more likely to have orgasm using this position than with just doing the missionary in the classic position.

There was 36 women that had never experienced orgasm using the classic missionary position that participated in a study. They were in a sexual workshop with their spouses that lasted for eight weeks. In these workshops they learned about ways that they could enhance their sexual communication skills. There was 19 members in the group that were asked to perform CAT during intimate moments with their partners. The other seventeen in the group were asked to masturbate to make them feel more sexually comfortable and capable of going through the sexual response cycle—excitement, plateau, orgasm, and resolution. Other studies have been done with 73% of women climaxing with the help of CAT.

The Clitty CAT is done by having the woman lie on her back, the man gets on top of her assuming the missionary position. At this point the man needs to move up a bit—over a bit to one side about two inches. His chest should be at her shoulders. The woman needs to bend her legs to a 45 degree angle. She then bends her hips upward aiding in the coital alignment. The base of the penis is constantly touching the woman's clitoris. Another way is have the woman wrap her legs around the man's thighs adding to the intimacy with more skin contact. The man can spice things up by doing a rocking or grinding motion instead of simply thrusting up and down. These motions can cause more friction that can lead to a climax. The CAT is a simple addition to sexual positions that can have astonishing benefits. It would be one great thing to add to your arsenal of sexual positions.

Chapter 2 – Rear Entry Penetration

The good old doggy style can sure feel good, but even this position can get boring if used too often. There are other more exciting sexual positions that go through the backdoor. What is good about these sexual positions is that they offer deep penetration. For those that are familiar with Yoga there is the "downward dog." There is also the "standing wheel barrow" sexual positions that enters from behind.

Standing Wheel Barrow
First the woman assumes the downward dog pose. This is bending over with both hands over the head and firmly planted on the floor while the legs are straight and the feet are planted on the floor as well. The shape of the woman should basically be like a triangle where the base of the triangle is the floor between her legs and the tip would be her buttocks. The woman needs to part her legs so that the man can position himself in behind her and in between her legs. He grabs her legs and lifts her up. She then wraps her legs around the man's waist for more support. He should be able to enter her now. This is a sexual position that is pretty hard to do for the woman. As she is baring her weight on her arms and hands. The guy needs to be strong enough that he can carry her and keep the balance. A good idea before adding this position is to limber up before attempting it. It can only be done for a short time due to its difficult position, the pleasure you and your partner will get will be well worth it.

Doggy Leg Lift

If you find that the "standing wheel barrow" position is too difficult no worries. You can still spice up the doggie style. With the standing wheel barrow the woman has to have both of her legs up, but the doggy leg lift only needs one up. On the bed the woman is on all-fours as she normally would be for the doggy style position. Then man then takes one of the woman's thighs and wraps it around his hip. He may need to do a bit of twisting about to make sure that both parties are in comfortable positions. Now he can enter her using thrusting, he can use one of his hands to touch the woman in other parts of her body as he thrusts into her. He can add to the stimulation of the woman by playing with her clitoris as he pumps from behind her.

Chapter 3 – Move Over to the Side Please

The sexual position called "Spork" is not about spanking, but that could certainly add some spice into the sexual encounter. It is also referred to as "scissoring" don't get freaked out it does not involve cutting anything off! It is not just about sex but about adding some creativity and a little flexibility into your sexual positions. Just like the utensil that combines the fork and the spoon to make a spork. Spooning is another classic sexual position and is considered one of the four basic sex positions with the other three being: doggy style, female superior position, and the missionary position.

In the spooning position the man lies right behind the woman while they both have their knees bent. He then takes the woman from behind while they are both in this lying position on their sides. The bodies can either be close to have that more intimate touching of each other or they can just be touching with only the pelvis. With just the pelvis touching this provides the man with better leverage for him to thrust deeper and harder. The woman can lift her upper leg to make the penetration easier for the man, this will also add more force on his thrusts.

This is a fun position that allows couples of have some close cuddling while getting it on. The guy can also allow his hands to explore his partners body, while he is thrusting from behind. He can grope her breasts and touch her clitoris giving her even more sexual arousal. The woman can also touch the male's scrotum during this coupling. When the man has his face close to the nape of the woman's neck he can kiss her neck and arouse her even more sexually.

The fork part of "sporking" involves the crossing of body parts that will make the couple look like a pair of scissors hence where the other name for it originates from. The couple start with the spoon position, then the man slowly moves down lower, the woman slowly lies down on her back. The man carries the woman's leg and places it on his shoulder. This allows for maximum penetration. The woman rises one of her legs allowing the male to slip in between her legs. Her left leg can be positioned between the man's knees. He should be at a 90 degree angle so that it will be easier for him to enter her. With the woman extending her legs like that she resembles a spork with her legs acting as the tines. The clitoris doesn't get much work in the spork position. It does allow the woman to fondle herself while the man is doing most of the work. While the woman has her leg on the man's shoulder this can give her a chance to pleasure herself while he is thrusting into her. Using the spork position is a good start into exploring new sexual positions.

You can learn to become creative in making up new sexual positions that you and your sexual partner both derive the most pleasure from. All you need is some creativity and flexibility and you will be well on your way to spicy things up in the bedroom!

Pretzel Dip or Camel Ride

The pretzel dip is another sexual position that should be included in every person's sexual repertoire. The pretzel dip also is known as the Camel style or Camel ride. This particular sexual position encourages clitoral contact and face-to-face sex making it one of the favorite sexual positions with both men and women.

To prepare for this sexual position the woman lies down on her right side, the man kneels and straddles her right leg. The woman then bends her left leg and curls it over the man's waist. The woman can also choose to leave her leg at her side if she does not want to wrap it around the man. This position will free her vagina making penetration easier for the man. The man can hold her raised leg to help keep her comfortable. This is a sexual position that allows for deep penetration similar when engaged in the doggie style position. The main difference is that you are able to have eye contact with your partner in this position. You can look into each other's eyes during this sexual position this will add to your bond with your partner and improve your relationship.

This position also allows the woman to enjoy the benefits of doggy style without getting pain or discomfort that many women experience during rear entry such as back aches. In this position the woman is on her side and can enjoy the deep penetrating sex more. The man can use his free hand to further pleasure the woman making things even more exciting for her. If he plays with her clitoris and strokes her other body parts such as her breasts this will help to enhance the woman's sexual experience.

Another good thing about the pretzel dip is that the man is able to control the rhythm. The man can also withdraw his penis and use it to play with the woman's clitoris, using it to tease her vagina with.

Chapter 4 – Movies Inspiring Sex On Staircases

Many couples today find that by watching movies that have sex scenes helps them to get in the mood for some fun sex in the bedroom. Watching movies with sex scenes can help give people ideas on how they can add some spice into their own sex lives. A good way to get some spark into your sex life might be to rent some movies that have some hot and steamy sex scenes and watch them with your sexual partner. These can be great aides in helping to plant that seed into you and your partner's mind for some great lovemaking. Two movies that have sex scenes in them that involve a staircase are *The Thomas Crown Affair, and A History of Violence.* Watching these films hot scenes on the stairs made one think that it looked pretty good. But you might one to keep in mind that sometimes looks can be deceiving as it is difficult to make love on such an uneven and hard surface. With this being said it is possible and it can be great!

Stairway to Heaven
First off this sexual position is not only for the stairs in your home or any other stairs for that matter. This position can also be achieved in a pool if it has stairs in it. Make sure that you have the pool all to yourself you do not want to run the risk of someone making a sex video of you do you? The woman should be sitting on the stair that aligns with the man's pelvis. The man's feet should be on the floor and his body leaning towards the woman. This is probably about the second or third step. While the woman is sitting she mover her arms behind her placing them on the stairs behind them. This is important because it helps to give support. She then opens her legs spreading them so that the man can enter her. The man will use his hands for support, but he may be strong enough to use only one hand and use the other to explore the woman's body adding to the overall

sensation. He should make his thrusts deep and wild to help her to reach orgasm. If you are doing this in a pool the thrusting motion will create small waves that can add to the woman's pleasure.

The Tabletop Position
A great sexy scene was in the movie *Pretty Woman* with Richard Gere and Julia Roberts when they are having a sexual tryst on top of a grand piano. The sexual position that they were using does not need a grand piano in order for you to perform it. Any high surface will do as long as the pelvis' of both parties align. It is a best if the surface is as high as the waist. The washing machine, dining room table, kitchen counter, your desk in your office these are just few suggestions where you might consider trying out this sexual position. The table top position is also known as the Torrid Table starts off with the woman sitting on the surface with her buttocks at the edge of surface. The woman can either spread her legs herself or let the man spread them.

The man then positions himself between the woman's legs. He is in a standing position. He then penetrates the woman's vagina and starts thrusting in and out of her. The woman might choose to lean back on her hands tilting her head back to help add to her sensations. She cannot see what is happening this way, she can only focus on the feeling of having sex. The same can be said if she lies down on her back. She may choose to wrap her legs around the guy, or have them hanging loose. There is more physical contact if she wraps her legs around the man. She may also decide to lean her body forward to be closer to the man. She may want to embrace him or wrap her arms around his neck. It will help to promote intimacy. The man could easily carry the woman from the table while her legs are wrapped around him and her arms are around his neck, from there he can place her on the bed. During this move he is still inside her. He can also continue to thrust into her in the leg lock position which involves him carrying the woman and thrusting into her without the use of a table or anything else.

Another variation of the Tabletop is the Lying Down Scissors. This involves the woman having her legs extended straight up parallel to the man, she then places her legs over one another. Her left leg will sit on his right shoulder and her right leg will sit on his left shoulder. In this position there is more clitoral stimulation because of the tighter feel. This is a position that both parties will enjoy.

The Sneak-A-Peek is another position that was derived from the Tabletop position. With this position the woman's forearms are flat on the surface behind her for support while her butt is hanging from the edge of surface. The man holds her feet and places them on top of his shoulders. In this position upper body strength is required as the man has to carry the woman. The man can see everything from where he is in this position. He can see her face, body, breasts, and her hot moist vagina. This is a great position that can help improve any couples sex life. Just by using other places besides the bedroom to have sex is a great way to add some spice into your sex life. You can do the Tabletop position anywhere in the house as long as the surface is waist-high. This is also the perfect position for the office desk or public place. This is a great position to keep in your repertoire just make sure to use some degree of caution when you are performing this position in a public place. Where there is a waist high surface there is a potential place for you to have some great sex using the Tabletop position.

Chapter 5 – Best Positions to Help You to Become Pregnant

If you are looking to increase the number in your family and are interested in becoming a parent, make sure that your partner is also open to becoming a parent. Do not try and get pregnant to someone that has no idea that you are trying to get pregnant. You want to have a child with a person that is also ready to become a parent. Do not try and get pregnant because you are desperate to try and stop your partner from leaving you. Getting pregnant is not the solution.

Adding new sexual positions to your repertoire will certainly improve your chance of keeping your relationship fun and interesting, but there is also other factors to consider when you are in a serious relationship. For one you should both be true to each other, and keep the lines of communication open. You need to be honest with your partner and talk to them about any issues that might bother you.   If you talk with them you both may be able to find a solution together. If there is no problem with your sex life and you are both happy with each other and have decided that it is time to have a baby then you should read on.

There are many couples that have trouble trying to conceive. Some couples will seek help from a fertility doctor while others rely on their ovulation period. Others may try praying to their gods for fertility. There is nothing wrong with taking these steps, but the best way to get pregnant is to get things happening as often as possible.   To help increase your chances of getting pregnant, try the sexual positions below.

Missionary

The classic man on top the missionary position is the most effective position to get pregnant. According to research it has found that the penis is closer to the cervix during the missionary position. MRI sans of copulating couples showed that the penis can go as far as the recess at the front of the uterus' opening.

Also many believe that the sperm travels down easier in the vagina of the woman when she is on her back. Once the deed is done the woman should lie on her back for about 15 minutes. There is no actual study that has been done to approve or disapprove that the missionary position increases chances for conception.

There was one study that was done one Intrauterine insemination or IUI treatment. In one group of women they were allowed to get up right after intercourse. The second group of women were asked to lie there afterwards for an additional 15 minutes after treatment. Those that kept lying on their backs for the additional 15 minutes had a 27% pregnancy rate compared to the group who got up right away that had an 18% pregnancy rate. This seems to prove that a woman's chances of becoming pregnant will increase.

Doggie Style

Another sex position that is said to help improve chances of becoming pregnant is doggie style. The tip of the man's penis is shown to be closest to the back of the woman's cervix during doggie style. In fact the penis reaches the recess of the cervix. You can also incorporate new positions with these old ones to keep your sex life spicy even when you are trying to conceive.

Tips for Wanna be Parents:

Studies have revealed that men who masturbate right after watching a pornographic films produce more semen, this will help to increase chances of getting woman pregnant. Another way to get a man excited so that he produces more sperm is to have longer periods of pre-sexual act—or foreplay.

If the man's sperm count is normal doing these things will only help increase semen production and allows more sperm to go through to the cervix. The wrong sexual position is not the reason for not getting pregnant. Anyone can get pregnant as long as the man ejaculates inside the woman and the sperm goes through to the cervix. There could be other underlying problems why you do not have a baby yet. The best thing you can do is to keep trying. With the help of the new different sexual positions described in this book getting pregnant is going to be so much fun for you and your partner!

Chapter 6 – The G-Spot

The G-spot has been recently documented in MRI scans and biopsies by medical doctors as a real part of a woman's anatomy. Now thanks to recent research we know that every woman is capable of experiencing more concentrated sexual pleasure—this includes powerful orgasms. We will guide you towards finding yours so you may lay back and enjoy the benefits that you will reap from your G-spot.

What is it exactly?
As far as the size of the G-spot there seems to be some disagreement; it may range from a quarter of an inch to a couple of inches along the wall of your vagina wall, about an inch or two past the opening of your vagina. Underneath it has highly sensitive tissue that when it is touched in the right way, this triggers sexual happiness, feelings of pleasure. Some women have described the sensations of the G-spot as being more intense than those they feel via a clitoral stimulation—more heated or warm, flushing feeling that seems to resonate deeply throughout their body.

The researchers have found that the G-spot is its own entity, analogous to an organ in the male body. It is known as the female prostrate because its tissue surrounds an area that produces chemicals that are similar to those made by the male prostrate, this is a gland that creates fluid to nourish sperm. Another similarity that the G-spot has with the male prostrate is that women state that they experience a wetness unlike they do with other types of stimulation. And some say that they ejaculate a clear odorless fluid upon orgasm.

Where to Locatc it
Start by lying back and relaxing—this can take some patience when trying to find your G-spot for the first time. Spread your legs and bending your knees, so that your vagina becomes open and accessible. With your palm facing up, insert two fingers inside, pressing your fingers against the center of the upper wall of your vagina. You are trying to locate a spongy, puckered, or slightly ridged area, like the roof of your mouth.

If you are still not able to find it try and think of a sexual fantasy while searching for it. When you are aroused your G-spot fills with fluid, making it swell and become larger. You will be able to locate it easier if you are turned on or aroused.

You may know that you have found it when you have the urge to pee all of a sudden. This happens because the G-spot is so close to the urethra, touching it often will trigger that urgent got to pee kind of feeling. There is no need to run to the washroom; it is a false alarm. After a few seconds this urge will pass and you will soon experience a kind of heated sensation that becomes more and more intense as you touch and stroke your G-spot area.

At the beginning do some experimenting on your own using different pressures with different speeds. Eventually you will find yourself getting closer and closer to having an orgasm. Don't hold back but allow yourself to experience a super intense G-spot orgasm before you show your sexual partner how they can take care of you down there.

Guiding Your Sexual Partner to Your G-spot
Remember how it took a bit of practice for you to train your sexual partner on how to pleasure your body's other pleasure points earlier in your relationship? Well expect the same with the G-spot as it is basically uncharted territory, especially for most men.

The easiest way to start your partner off is to have them gently slip one or two fingers inside your vagina, then have them softly feel along your upper vaginal wall. If your partner is having trouble finding your G-spot, encourage them to touch and kiss your in other areas of your body to help to sexually arose you, remember your G-spot will stand out when you are aroused making it easier to find.

You can also try to put some pillows under your butt, this will help to open your vagina more and give your partner easier access. When your partner has located the spot ask them to massage it in slow gentle circles. You might want to try different styles of caresses such as doing figure eights or doing a rapid succession of pulses. Your G-spot can take a lot of pressure, so you may want to ask him to press harder on it.

One G-spot technique that you should try is called tapping. Have your partner use the tip of their finger to tap firmly and repeatedly on your G-spot. When you use this technique it is like your G-spot is getting touched for the first time over and over again and this can lead to an explosive orgasm.

Sexual Positions that Increase G-spot Pleasure

When woman are on top this is a G-spot winner in sexual positions. When you are sitting on top of a penis and leaning slightly back their penis is naturally resting against your upper vaginal wall. The slightest thrusting can stimulate your G-spot. You can be in control on top and you can position your partner's penis so that it is hitting your G-spot.

Doggie-style also offers maximum access, especially if you are lying on your stomach with your legs spread slightly. When you are on your stomach and have your legs spread slightly this helps to sandwich the vagina walls so that your partner's penis will come in contact with your G-spot.

It can also be stimulated in the missionary position, just keep your knees bent and feet resting flat on the bed, raise your pelvis by putting some pillows under your butt, this will give the penis of your partner access to your upper vaginal wall. You will then be able to feel your G-spot being stimulated with each back and forth thrust.

Trick for Ultimate G-spot Bliss

The blended orgasm tops them all when it comes to having an intense orgasm. To experience this you combine the G-spot stimulation with the stimulating of your clitoris, working your way to a double your pleasure orgasm. The nerves of the G-spot and the clitoris are very close so reaching the peak via the two types of touching at the same time is about as intense as you are going to get.

To experience a blended orgasm during foreplay you can get your partner to massage your clitoris with one hands fingers while he has the other hands fingers inside your vagina stimulating your G-spot. As you become more excited lift your pelvis so that you are thrusting against his hand. Ask your partner to flick your clitoris with their tongue also.

Another blended orgasm position is doggie-style, where you kneel low on your knees and forearms and put your pelvis lifted off the bed so he can reach your clitoris or you can to stimulate it. You can also have him thrust a bit then have him stop to stimulate your clitoris.

Your best bet for the blended orgasm is to use the woman-on-top position. You can angle your body in such a way so that his penis is rubbing against your G-spot then have him play with your clitoris at the same time.

Make sure to encourage him to continue to pleasure you inside and outside pleasure zones until you finally surrender to orgasm. You will not only enjoy the deep physical pleasure with your sexual partner but you will build a deep emotional connection with them too.

Boosting the Power of Your G-spot
Just like many things practice makes perfect, this is also true when it comes to your G-spot. The more that you incorporate it into your sexual repertoire the easier it is going to be for you to reach G-spot nirvana.

You can deepen the sensations that you have by regularly doing Kegel exercises. These are when you contract your pubococcygeus muscles, giving you a tighter grip during intercourse that helps to add pleasure to your G-spot.

The way to do these is to zero in on the muscle in your pelvis that can stop the flow of urine. Squeeze as tight as you can, and hold for five seconds, then release. You can do this exercise during downtime such as sitting in traffic, multiple times throughout the day. If you do ten minutes of Kegels a day that should make your G-spot more responsive.

Conclusion

I hope that you and your partner will enjoy trying out the assortment of sexual positions offered in my book. I am sure that you will find that they are going to add some great spice and a boost to your love life. Try and get creative in the bedroom add some personal swings to these sexual positions and really make your lover beg for more!

If you enjoyed reading my book and found it helpful I would appreciate it if you could leave a small review at Amazon. Thanks again for your support in downloading my book!